WHY YOU'RE FAT & SICK
AND HOW TO FIX IT!

OUR TOP 10 TIPS TO MAKE
YOU LEAN, SEXY, & HEALTHY!

By: Christopher & Stacy Mitchell

www.ChangeYourLifeOvernight.com

WHY YOU'RE FAT & SICK AND HOW TO FIX IT! OUR TOP 10 TIPS TO MAKE YOU LEAN, SEXY, & HEALTHY!

Copyright © 2017 Christopher Mitchell

ISBN-13: 978-1543180305

ISBN-10: 1543180302

Printed In The United States Of America.

TABLE OF CONTENTS:

Let us teach you how to become a Self-Published Author in record time! It's fast, cheap, and simple! We'll send you all our best Tips, Facts, & Statistics **ABSOLUTELY FREE**! The only thing you need to do is submit your name and email address right here:

www.ChangeYourLifeOvernight.com

Chapter One:

Who Are We?

Christopher & Stacy Mitchell are a husband and wife team that have 36 years of combined experience in the Health, Fitness, & Medical industries.

For over 21 years Christopher was a Champion Competitive Bodybuilder, a Fitness Magazine Cover Model, a Professional Nutritionist, as well as a Certified Personal Trainer. He practices what he preaches and has changed thousands of people's lives for the better through his knowledge and wisdom of exercise, nutrition, and supplementation.

Christopher has helped people all over the world lose weight, increase strength, build muscle, and eliminate cancer, diabetes, multiple sclerosis, and arthritis to name just a few.

For over 15 years Stacy was a Registered Nurse in the ER at Ohio State University Medical Center. While there, she witnessed some of the most gruesome things that a person could ever see.

She took care of diabetics, cancer patients, rape victims, people with aids, allergies, anorexia, arthritis, autism, bipolar disorder, bulimia, dementia, fibromyalgia, and every other disease you can imagine. She also cared for little children who had been molested, and people who had body parts blown off by gun shot.

She has seen it all. However, most of the health problems she witnessed in the emergency room could have easily been prevented had the people taken better care of their health.

Christopher and Stacy have seen the effects of what happens to a person when they don't take care of their health, and they've also cured people after they destroyed their health. So, if you're still alive it's not too late for you to turn your health around. Everything written in this book is documented facts. Nothing is based on their opinions.

Christopher and Stacy don't smoke, drink, or do any drugs whatsoever. They haven't got the flu, been sick, or even been to a Doctor in many years. The knowledge they're going to share with you in this book can turn your life around in no time at all. If you're willing to accept the information as true, and then walk it out by making some changes in your daily lifestyle, you can live in perfect health. However, if you want your health to change, you have to be willing to make some changes.

Chapter Two:

Why You're Fat & Sick.

Instead of candy coating things let's just get straight to the truth! The reason why you're fat and sick is because of what YOU put inside of your body every single day. If you eat sugar you're poisoning your health. If you eat dairy you're poisoning your health. If you eat gluten you're poisoning your health. If you eat anything that is NOT 100% organic you're poisoning your health. If you drink alcohol you're poisoning your health. If you use any kind of tobacco you're poisoning your health. If you take ANY type of pharmaceutical drug whatsoever you're poisoning your health. If you're fat and sick like 98% of the population is YOU have to take responsibility and admit that it's YOUR fault. You caused it! Period!

We as Americans would rather have convenience than good health. We would rather buy our dinner at the McDonald's drive thru window than go home and cook a healthy, organic meal. We would rather go out and poison ourselves at happy hour to please our friends than telling them no so we can live longer. We would rather go out to eat every single day at lunch with our coworkers than to prepare our food at home ahead of time. We would rather buy a BIG GULP soda at the gas station than a bottle of water. These actions that people make every single day is why they're fat and sick. Until you change your daily habits you will continue to be fat and sick. And guess what? The fatter and sicker you get brings you that much closer to dying prematurely. You're committing suicide! Suicide is the #1 way that people die in America. You probably never would have thought you would commit suicide, but that's what you're doing every time you put something poisonous inside of your body. It will catch up with you. Every single disease in the world is caused by what people put inside of their body. That's the truth!

If you smoke cigarettes you will get cancer. If you take prescription drugs you will get side effects. If you continue to eat sugar you will get fatter, and possibly diabetes. If you get the flu shot you will get the flu. If you get chemo and radiation you will get weak and lose your hair, and possibly die. It's time to wake up! When did Americans become so stupid? It's time to stop committing suicide by poisoning yourself every single day. It will catch up with you and you will die prematurely.

www.Dictionary.com says these are the definitions of these two words:

Fat: having too much flabby tissue.

Sick: afflicted with ill health or disease.

According to those definitions about 98% of the population is fat and sick. It's sad, but very true. In order to get fat and sick is simply a matter of self-disrespect. The ONLY way to get fat and sick is by what you put inside of your body. That means a person is putting garbage inside of their body in order to become fat and sick. To put garbage inside of your body means you don't respect yourself. Otherwise, why in the world would you put toxic garbage inside of yourself? You're destroying your body. You're destroying your health. You're committing suicide!

Did you know that being fat actually causes you to be sick? It does. Let us prove it to you. Being fat weakens your immune system. Fat people have suppressed and broken immune systems. Fat people are more prone to infections. Layers of bodyfat prevent healing from occurring. Fat people are more susceptible to autoimmune disorders like diabetes, Crohn's disease, multiple sclerosis, and rheumatoid arthritis. Fat people get the flu and pneumonia more often than people who have lower bodyfat levels. Fat people are also prone to sleep apnea because they have a harder time breathing. Fat people are usually depressed, and depression causes people to binge eat, which only makes them fatter and sicker. Fat people have a digestive system that is out of whack and this causes constipation, bloating, and acid reflux. Fat people have a slow metabolism, which causes low energy and fatigue.

So, as you can clearly see, it's a fact that being fat causes all kinds of illness, sickness, and disease. A person could eliminate a lot of their sickness just by losing weight. Being a Professional Nutritionist and Certified Personal Trainer, Christopher is a master at teaching people how to lose weight. The first book that he wrote actually teaches people how to lose weight FAST! The book is titled:

HOW TO LOSE WEIGHT WITH INTERMITTENT FASTING! It will teach you how to lose up to 30 pounds in 30 days. You can buy the book on Amazon, or by clicking this link: www.ChangeYourLifeOvernight.com

Chapter Three:

Sugar.

What exactly is sugar? Sugar is a mixture of dextrose and fructose that are contained in various foods and drinks. Dextrose and fructose are both monosaccharides, known as simple sugars. The primary difference between them is how your body metabolizes them. The simple sugars can combine to form more complex sugars like the disaccharide sucralose, which is one half glucose and one half fructose. Sucralose (Splenda) is not actual sugar, despite its name. However, it's a chlorinated artificial sweetener in line with aspartame and it has detrimental side effects to your long term health. Nothing good can come from consuming sugar. If you decide to eat or drink sugar you will absolutely suffer the consequences.

Sugar makes people fat and sick! Period. Sugar is more addictive than cocaine! If I asked you, would you like some cocaine? You would probably respond absolutely not! Well then, why in the world would you like some sugar? Sugar is worse on your health than cocaine!

The average American consumes more than 150 pounds of sugar per year. Sugar is toxic, addicting, and deadly! Most of the parents in the world would never even consider giving their kids cocaine, but for some reason they have no problem giving their kids sugar, which is even more addicting. Parents are terrible role models for their children by allowing them to consume sugar.

Isn't is obvious why Americans are so fat and sick? We consume more sugar than any other country in the world. Sugar is one of the deadliest killers we have in the world today. Consumption of foods containing sugar costs Americans over $54 BILLION per year in dental bills. Sugar is destroying people's teeth at an alarming rate. Do you know that 92% of American adults have tooth decay? Do you know that the ONLY cause of tooth decay is sugar? It's true!

Sugar is bad for your health in every area, both internally and externally. It even increases the aging process. After sugar hits your bloodstream it ends up attaching itself to proteins in a process called glycation. These new molecular structures contribute to the loss of elasticity found in aging body tissues. This includes everything from your skin, to your organs and arteries. The more sugar circulating in your bloodstream means the faster your health will deteriorate.

Let us give you just a few of the health problems that can be caused by consuming sugar:

-Cancer

-Obesity

-Arthritis

-Allergies

-Diabetes

-Dementia

-Headaches

-Depression

-Tooth Decay

-Liver Disease

-Inflammation

-Hypertension

-Heart Attacks

-Heart Disease

-Kidney Disease

-Alzheimer's Disease.

The biggest problem from consuming sugar is of course: **DEATH!**

Consuming sugar is one of the very worst things you could ever do to your health, and is guaranteed to make you fat, sick, and **DIE**. If you continue to consume sugar you will continue to be fat and sick, and you will eventually **DIE** from the side effects. If you want to become lean, sexy, and healthy you absolutely must eliminate sugar from your life. This is 100% non-negotiable!

Chapter Four:

Dairy.

What exactly is dairy? Dairy is a food product made from the milk of mammals. Human beings were never meant to consume this crap. It's poisonous to your health and will definitely make you fat and sick.

The majority of dairy products in America come from dairy farmers who inject their cows with genetically engineered bovine growth hormone. Dairy farmers inject their cows with this drug to increase milk production. This forces the cows to produce more milk than they ever could naturally. This un-natural increase in milk production leads to the cows having their udders infected. An infected udder is then treated with more drugs known as antibiotics. These unhealthy antibiotics then make their way into the dairy products that you consume, which ends up making you fat and sick. Are you starting to see why dairy is so bad for you now?

Dairy is highly acidic. Milk is rich in natural acids that cause calcium deposits to build up and potentially cause arthritis and inflammation inside the human body. Dairy is one of the hardest products to digest, and also causes many different types of disease. It also increases aging.

As superficial as it might seem, your skin's health is just as important as any other aspect of your health. Why? Because it shows how healthy the inside of your body is. Your skin is the largest organ on your body and whatever the internal body can't get rid of the skin will try to do itself. This is especially true when it comes to the liver and digestive system having a hard time with internal wastes that can't be properly removed. When you consume dairy the skin usually takes a major hit. You'll see this through acne, redness, and splotchy skin. Many people notice huge improvements to their skin the first few days they go without dairy. This is because the inside of the body is better able to clean itself out and the skin isn't left to do all the work.

Dairy can also cause gut damage due to the way it inflames the gut lining. Dairy causes leaky gut syndrome like nothing else. Having a leaky gut causes autoimmune diseases and other health issues. Dairy will also disturb your digestive system and cause bloating, constipation, diarrhea, and even irritable bowel syndrome. People who suffer from serious disorders such as Crohn's disease find that once they eliminate dairy from their diets they naturally become healed.

Dairy has been found to be a leading cause of prostate, breast, testicular, and colon cancer. Dairy is not healthy and you shouldn't consume it. A plant based diet free from dairy has been found to be one of the best ways to prevent cancer and other diseases.

The main carbohydrate in dairy is lactose. This is a sugar that is made from the two simple sugars glucose and galactose. When we were infants our bodies produced a digestive enzyme called lactase. This breaks down lactose from mother's milk. However, many people lose the ability to do this when they become adults. In fact, about 75% of the world's population is unable to break down lactose as adults. This is called lactose intolerance. People who are lactose intolerant have digestive symptoms when they consume dairy products. This includes nausea, vomiting, and diarrhea. Some people are also allergic to the protein in milk.

Dairy production is also very cruel to both baby and adult cows. Baby calves are taken away from their mothers at birth. Mother cows will cry and search for their calves after they've been separated. While female calves are either slaughtered, or kept alive only to produce milk, male calves are chained up in tiny stalls and raised for veal. Since it's unprofitable for dairy farmers to keep dairy cows alive once their milk production declines, these cows are slaughtered once they reach 5 or 6 years old, even though their normal life span exceeds 20 years. When you consume dairy you're being cruel to cows, and poisoning yourself.

Let us give you just a few of the health problems that can be caused by consuming dairy:

-Acne

-Cancer

-Obesity

-Arthritis

-Allergies

-Diabetes

-Diarrhea

-Flatulence

-Headaches

-Tooth Decay

-Osteoporosis

-Inflammation

-Heart Disease

-Lactose Intolerance

-Forms A Lot Of Mucus

-Cardiovascular Disease

-Irritable Bowel Syndrome

-Increased Mortality Risk By 93%

The biggest problem from consuming dairy is of course: **DEATH!**

Consuming dairy is one of the very worst things you could ever do to your health, and is guaranteed to make you fat, sick, and **DIE**. If you continue to consume dairy you will continue to be fat and sick, and you will eventually **DIE** from the side effects. If you want to become lean, sexy, and healthy you absolutely must eliminate dairy from your life. This is 100% non-negotiable!

Chapter Five:

Wheat.

What exactly is wheat? Wheat is a cereal grain. Wheat is loaded with gluten. Gluten is the main protein found in wheat, rye, spelt and barley. The problem with consuming wheat is that people are unable to properly digest the gluten in it. Your immune system recognizes gluten proteins in the digestive tract, thinks they're foreign invaders, and mounts an attack against the gluten, and the digestive wall itself. Gluten can damage the intestinal lining, and cause symptoms like pain, anemia, bloating, diarrhea, and tiredness.

Wheat products get digested quickly, which leads to large spikes in your blood sugar levels. These large spikes are followed by rapid drops, which increase hunger and cravings. This will make a person fat and sick. Wheat isn't nutritious compared to other real foods like meats and vegetables. Wheat also contains substances that steal nutrients from other foods. Wheat doesn't contain all the essential amino acids in the right ratios, and is therefore not a very good source of protein for human beings. Wheat contains a substance called phytic acid, which can reduce absorption of important minerals.

Studies show that wheat consumption is associated with serious brain disorders. Cerebellar ataxia is a motor disturbance caused by lesions in the cerebellum which is a part of the brain that controls motor functions. This disease can be caused by gluten consumption. It's called gluten ataxia and involves an autoimmune attack on the cerebellum. Schizophrenia is a serious mental disorder. There are strong statistical associations between celiac disease, gluten sensitivity, and schizophrenia. Many schizophrenic individuals have antibodies against gluten in their bloodstream. Autism and epilepsy can also be caused by gluten sensitivity. Given that there's no actual benefit to eating wheat, I would prefer to be on the safe side and simply avoid it.

When gluten proteins are broken down in a test tube the peptides they form are able to stimulate opioid receptors. These peptides are called gluten exorphins. Opioid receptors are the receptors in the brain that are stimulated by drugs like heroin and morphine. When you eat gluten it gets broken down into these opioid peptides, which then travels into your blood, and eventually into your brain where they cause addiction to wheat.

You probably didn't know that consuming wheat causes over 200 different health issues did you? This is absolutely insane! Let us give you just a few of the health problems that can be caused by consuming wheat:

-Cancer

-Autism

-Asthma

-Obesity

-Seizures

-Epilepsy

-Diarrhea

-Psoriasis

-Diabetes

-Infertility

-Dementia

-Miscarriage

-Inflammation

-Kidney Stones

-Schizophrenia

-Celiac Disease

-Food Allergies

-Down Syndrome

-Hyperthyroidism

-Multiple Sclerosis

-Migraine Headaches

-Cardiovascular Disease

-Coronary Artery Disease

-Irritable Bowel Syndrome

The biggest problem from eating wheat is of course: **DEATH!**

Consuming wheat is one of the very worst things you could ever do to your health, and is guaranteed to make you fat, sick, and **DIE**. If you continue to eat wheat you will continue to be fat and sick, and you will eventually **DIE** from the side effects. If you want to become lean, sexy, and healthy you absolutely must eliminate wheat from your life. This is 100% non-negotiable!

Chapter Six:

HFCS.

What exactly is HFCS? HFCS is the abbreviated letters for the words: **High Fructose Corn Syrup**. HFCS is a commonly known sweetener derived from cornstarch that food and drink manufacturers put inside of their products. This stuff is not only making you fat and sick, but it is downright killing you! HFCS is in almost every single type of product in the world nowadays!

One 20 ounce soda sweetened with HFCS contains a whopping 17 teaspoons of sugar. The average teenager consumes two of these soda beverages per day. The average adult consumes even more. So, that means Americans are consuming a bare minimum of 34 teaspoons of sugar every single day. Our ancestors consumed on average 20 teaspoons of sugar per year. That's a HUGE difference! I personally consume less than 1 teaspoon of sugar per day.

Products containing HFCS are sweeter and cheaper than products made with real cane sugar. This allowed the average soda size to increase from 8 ounces to 20 ounces without any extra costs to the manufacturers, but a huge increase in costs for humans by increased obesity, diabetes, and many other serious diseases all in the name of GREED! People are committing murder every single day in the United States and they could care less as long as they get richer. It's time for you to wake up!

HFCS has been proven to literally punch holes in the intestinal lining allowing nasty byproducts of toxic gut bacteria and partially digested food proteins to enter your blood stream and trigger the inflammation that is at the root of every single disease.

A researcher from the FDA asked corn producers to ship a barrel of HFCS to her in order to test for contaminants. Her repeated requests were refused until she claimed she represented a newly created soft drink company. She was then promptly shipped a big vat of high fructose corn syrup that was used as part of the study that showed large toxic levels of mercury.

If you see high fructose corn syrup on the label of any product it is 100% pure poison. It is completely void of any healthy fiber, vitamins, minerals, phytonutrients, and antioxidants that your body desperately needs.

In America, medical bills to treat diseases associated with obesity are more than $200 billion per year. The majority of the obesity problem is because of food additives like HFCS. Food companies love putting this dangerous poison in their products because it's very cheap to manufacture, and allows them to make huge profit margins.

Another reason to avoid HFCS is because it is derived from genetically modified corn. That means it was developed in a lab, not grown and milled in the healthy, rich soil of the earth. Anytime you put something in your mouth that was developed in a laboratory you are guaranteed to be poisoning yourself.

The Center for Disease Control and Prevention data on weight gain illustrates that our obesity epidemic accelerated dramatically after genetically modified organism foods were introduced in the early 1990s. It's estimated that more than 80% of everything eaten in the United States today is genetically altered in a lab. This perfectly explains why Americans are so fat and sick. They're getting absolutely zero nutrition whatsoever!

Let us give you just a few of the health problems that can be caused by consuming HFCS:

-Cancer

-Obesity

-Arthritis

-Allergies

-Diabetes

-Dementia

-Headaches

-Depression

-Tooth Decay

-Liver Disease

-Inflammation

-Hypertension

-Heart Attacks

-Heart Disease

-Kidney Disease

-Alzheimer's Disease

-Leaky Gut Syndrome

The biggest problem from consuming HFCS is of course: **DEATH!**

Consuming HFCS is one of the very worst things you could ever do to your health, and is guaranteed to make you fat, sick, and **DIE**. If you continue to consume HFCS you will continue to be fat and sick, and you will eventually **DIE** from the side effects. If you want to become lean, sexy, and healthy you absolutely must eliminate HFCS from your life. This is 100% non-negotiable!

Chapter Seven:

Drugs.

What are drugs? More specifically, pharmaceutical drugs? Since I'm the one writing this book I'm going to give you my personal definition of what Pharmaceutical drugs are. Pharmaceutical drugs are one of the biggest scams the world has ever seen. Pharmaceutical drugs do nothing but cause people to get fat, sick, and believe it or not, die. That's the 100% absolute truth! I hope you're open minded enough to accept that, or at least investigate it to find out the truth for yourself.

Most people in the world have a Doctor that introduces them to pharmaceutical drugs. The Doctor told them that if they didn't take a specific pharmaceutical drug they would probably die. This mental brainwashing is purely selfish and demonic. Since a Doctor is looked at as an authority figure, and someone who is influential in the community people simply believe what a Doctor says without doing any research of their own to see if the Doctor might be wrong, which they are A LOT.

The word pharmaceutical came from the Greek word pharmakeia. Do you know what pharmakeia means?

Pharmakeia: witchcraft, magic, the use of spells often involving drugs.

It is a fact that witchcraft and magic in the Greek world often involved the use of drugs. Pharmaceutical drugs were created by Satan, the devil. Satan is using pharmaceutical drugs to destroy human beings. Satan is the king of lies, and to have a Doctor tell you that you must take a bunch of pharmaceutical drugs is a downright lie from the pit of hell. Satan has brain washed almost everyone into believing that we must take pharmaceutical drugs. This is sorcery, witchcraft, and demonic. This should make you start to think twice before putting pharmaceutical drugs inside your body.

Most people would never even think about snorting cocaine, smoking crack, or injecting heroine into their body, but these same people have no problem putting deadly pharmaceutical drugs inside of their body. People have been brain washed. Pharmaceutical drugs are demonic and deadly! In The Holy Bible it says in 2 Corinthians 2:11- **in order that Satan might not outwit us. For we are not unaware of his schemes**.

Unfortunately, Satan has outwitted most of the Americans today. Pharmakeia has a symbol associated with it, and that symbol is "Rx". People in the world today know that the symbol "Rx" means prescription drugs. This may surprise you, but the "Rx" symbol is actually the Eye of Horus, the identifying mark of Horus-Jupiter-Zeus! This also compares to the glowing capstone of the pyramid on the back of the one dollar bill.

If you understand the meaning of symbols, then you know the "Rx" symbol as the Eye of Horus links pharmaceutical drugs to the mark of the Beast ploy. There is nothing ambiguous about this connection because anything identified with such a mark means what all similar symbols mean. The "Rx" symbol, and the spell inducing drug scheme it represents exist only to facilitate the mark of the beast. The health care industry has been, and continues to be signaled by the secret elite agencies as the primary sector in which the mark of the best will be introduced to the world.

The "Rx" symbol also has another interpretation that provides an interesting perspective. "Rx" is an abbreviation for the Latin word "recipere", which means "take". This is an expression of a command to receive the drug being offered. The interpretation of "Rx" as "recipere" acknowledges the symbol as a command to receive the pharmakeia.

This compares to the inducement inherent in the name "PositiveId", the implantable microchip family of companies recently renamed from Verichip. PositiveId is equivalent to accepting the mark of the beast.

These two inducements "take" and "accept the mark" have already teamed up with the implantable microchip functioning as a "Rx" delivery system, and as a means of linking the chipped person to their medical records. This includes their actual prescriptions. Don't take my word for this. Research this for yourself, just like I encourage you to start researching everything that you put inside of your body.

Pharmaceutical drugs induce changes in your body chemistry. These effect your body's ability to function. Drugs influence how you feel, think and act. Every pharmaceutical drug in the world has negative side effects. These side effects control a person's brain and physical capabilities. If a Demon, ooops, I mean if a Doctor prescribes you a pharmaceutical drug you will get side effects. These side effects change your physical body composition, and then the Doctor gives you a prescription for another pharmaceutical drug to combat the negative side effects from the first drug. This continues until the side effects end your life. Had you never taken that first demon, I mean drug, you would be able to live a long, happy, and healthy lifestyle, the exact opposite of what Satan wants for you. Because you believed the Doctor without first educating yourself to see if what he said was true, the Doctor has now programmed you mentally to do whatever he tells you to. He has deceived you, just like Satan deceived Adam and Eve in The Garden Of Eden.

My mom died at the very young age of 35 years old because she listened to a demon, I mean Doctor. She was perfectly healthy, but then a Doctor told her she MUST start chemo and radiation immediately. Without getting a second opinion, or doing any research on her own, she simply told the Doctor ok. She did exactly what he told her to. Within a couple of months she was dead! I'm now 3 years older than my mom was when she died. I feel like my life is just beginning. I can't possibly even imagine dying when I was 35 years old. My wife and I are perfectly healthy. We have never taken prescription drugs, we never get sick, we haven't been to a Doctor in many years, and we don't even have health insurance. We don't need it!

What I'm sharing with you in this book will change your life forever if you'll simply do what I'm teaching. There is no reason whatsoever to ever take a pharmaceutical drug. You are killing yourself if you do.

Over two million people die every single year from the side effects of pharmaceutical drugs. This isn't my opinion, but documented fact. If you take pharmaceutical drugs you have got to be mentally insane, especially if you continue to take them after reading this book. I'm not going to apologize for saying this. I'm telling you the truth because I'm trying to save your life.

The pharmaceutical industry makes BILLIONS of dollars in profits every single year at the expense of millions of people dying. Eli Lilly, a major pharmaceutical company made $36 Billion from Zyprexa in just one year.

Pharmaceutical companies pay out Billions of dollars in lawsuits every single year from people dying, but for some reason these stories never seem to reach the media.

Let us give you just a few of the health problems that are caused by taking pharmaceutical drugs:

-Cancer

-Seizures

-Paranoia

-Depression

-Liver Failure

-Malnutrition

-Memory Loss

-Brain Damage

-Kidney Failure

-Mental Disorder

-Chronic Insomnia

-Respiratory Failure

-Physical Dependence

-Cardiovascular Disease

-Psychological Addiction

-Loss Of Cognitive Function

The biggest problem from taking pharmaceutical drugs is of course: **DEATH!**

Taking pharmaceutical drugs is one of the very worst things you could ever do to your health, and is guaranteed to make you fat, sick, and **DIE**. If you continue to take pharmaceutical drugs you will continue to be fat and sick, and you will eventually **DIE** from the side effects. If you want to become lean, sexy, and healthy you absolutely must eliminate pharmaceutical drugs from your life. This is 100% non-negotiable!

Chapter Eight:

Alcohol.

What is alcohol? Alcohol (ethanol) is a colorless, volatile, flammable liquid that is produced by the natural fermentation of sugars, and is the main ingredient found in beer, wine, and spirits that causes drunkenness. Alcohol is also used as an industrial solvent and as fuel.

Did you just see that? Alcohol is volatile? Alcohol is flammable? Alcohol is produced from sugar? Alcohol is used as an industrial solvent and fuel? Are you kidding me? And yet, people still drink this crap? No wonder why they're fat and sick! If you're willing to drink an ingredient that is used in an industrial solvent and in fuel, then you deserve to be fat and sick.

Pay attention the next time you pump gas in your car. On the actual pump it will clearly say: contains 10% ethanol. People are drinking the same exact stuff that they put in their gas tank. That is disgusting, and should be downright illegal!

Alcohol is classed as a sedative hypnotic drug, which means it acts to depress the central nervous system. Alcohol can act as a stimulant, inducing feelings of euphoria and talkativeness, and drinking a lot of alcohol can lead to drowsiness, respiratory failure, coma, and even death. Alcohol has effects on every organ in the body. When you drink alcohol it's absorbed into your bloodstream and gets distributed throughout your entire body. Doesn't that just make you want to go out and get drunk right now?

Alcohol consumption causes physical and emotional changes that will do great harm to your body. Drinking alcohol regularly will put your health in serious jeopardy, and shorten your life span. Drinking alcohol will cause the pancreas to produce toxic substances that interfere with proper functioning. The resulting inflammation is called pancreatitis, a serious problem that can destroy the pancreas. The most frequent cause of pancreatitis is consuming alcohol.

The job of the liver is to break down harmful substances, including alcohol. Drinking alcohol can cause hepatitis which can lead to the development of jaundice. Chronic liver inflammation can lead to severe scarring known as cirrhosis. This formation of scar tissue can destroy the liver. Liver disease is a life threatening disease.

One of the first signs of alcohol in your system is a change in behavior. Alcohol travels through the body easily. It can quickly reach many parts of your body, including your brain, and your central nervous system. That can make it harder to talk, causing slurred speech, which is a sign that someone has had too much alcohol to drink. It can also affect coordination, interfering with the ability to walk. Damage to your nervous system can result in pain, numbness, and abnormal sensations in your feet and hands.

Consuming alcohol can wreak havoc on your digestive system all the way from your mouth to your colon. Even a single night of drinking alcohol can injure parts of your digestive tract. Alcohol consumption can damage the salivary glands, irritate the mouth, lead to gum disease, tooth decay, and even tooth loss. Drinking alcohol can cause ulcers in the esophagus, acid reflux, and heartburn. Stomach ulcers and inflammation of the stomach lining can occur.

Erectile dysfunction is a common side effect of alcohol consumption in men. It can also inhibit hormone production, affect testicular function, and cause infertility. Women who consume alcohol can stop menstruating and become infertile. It can increase her risk of miscarriage, premature delivery, and stillbirth. If a woman does give birth to a baby while having alcohol in her system the baby can have physical abnormalities, learning difficulties, and emotional problems.

Drinking alcohol regularly makes it harder for your body to produce new bone. Consuming alcohol also puts you at increased risk of osteoporosis, and bone fractures. Muscles also become prone to weakness, have cramps, and even atrophy. Alcohol weakens your immune system making it harder for you to fight off germs, viruses, and all types of different illnesses. Alcohol drinkers are more likely to get pneumonia, tuberculosis, and cancer compared to the general population as well.

We also know what can happen when someone drinks alcohol, and then decides to drive a motor vehicle while they're intoxicated. Innocent lives are lost all because of a selfish drinker. Over 10,000 people die every single year in America because of an intoxicated driver. Of all the traffic related deaths in The United States each year, 31% of them are caused from alcohol consumption.

Let us give you just a few of the health problems that are caused by consuming alcohol:

-Coma

-Stroke

-Nausea

-Anxiety

-Jaundice

-Cirrhosis

-Hepatitis

-Dementia

-Confusion

-Drowsiness

-Heart Attack

-Malnutrition

-Hypothermia

-Inflammation

-Hyperglycemia

-Respiratory Failure

-Erectile Dysfunction

The biggest problem from drinking alcohol is of course: **DEATH!**

Consuming alcohol is one of the very worst things you could ever do to your health, and is guaranteed to make you fat, sick, and **DIE**. If you continue to consume alcohol you will continue to be fat and sick, and you will eventually **DIE** from the side effects. If you want to become lean, sexy, and healthy you absolutely must eliminate alcohol from your life. This is 100% non-negotiable!

Chapter Nine:

Tobacco.

What is tobacco? Tobacco is a green, leafy plant that is filled with nicotine. After tobacco is picked it is then dried, ground up, and used in different ways. It can be smoked in a pipe, cigar, or cigarette. It can also be chewed, or sniffed through the nose.

Nicotine is only one of more than 4,000 chemicals in tobacco. Nicotine is the chemical that makes tobacco addicting. Once you smoke, chew, or sniff tobacco, nicotine goes into your bloodstream and your body starts to crave more. The nicotine in tobacco makes it a drug. This means that when you use tobacco it changes your body in different ways. Because nicotine is a stimulant it speeds up your nervous system, which makes you feel like you have more energy. It also makes your heart beat faster and raises your blood pressure. Everyone in the entire world knows that tobacco kills you. So, why does the government allow it to be sold? That's an obvious reason- MONEY!

The tobacco industry is big business. Tobacco companies make so much money because the manufacturing costs are so low. The making of cigarettes is almost completely automated. Manufacturing cigarettes is done mostly by machines. This eliminates the costs of having to pay employees. Machines crush tobacco leaves. Machines clean tobacco leaves. Machines add in the nicotine. Machines also roll cigarettes, put on the filters, cut them to length, and then package them. The tobacco industry is done almost entirely by machines. This keeps the overhead low, and the profit margins high. Let me give you some facts about the immoral, greedy tobacco industry:

-There are approximately 20 states in America that grow tobacco.

-North Carolina, Kentucky, and Georgia account for nearly 80% of the tobacco production in America.

-The United States is the 4th largest tobacco producing country in the world, following China, India, and Brazil.

-Tobacco farms in the United States produce around 800 million pounds of tobacco per year.

-In 2014, tobacco companies spent more than $9 billion marketing cigarettes and smokeless tobacco in the United States. This amount equals around $25 million per day, or about $1 million per hour.

-During 2015, more than 264 billion cigarettes were sold in America.

-Philip Morris USA, Reynolds American Inc, ITG Brands, and Liggett, are the four biggest sellers of cigarettes in America. In 2015, these four companies accounted for about 91% of all the cigarettes sold in the United States.

-If a person smokes just one pack of cigarettes per day they will spend over $2,000 per year on the habit.

-Smoking related illnesses in the United States costs more than $300 billion every year.

-Cigarette smoking causes more than 480,000 deaths every single year in the United States. One out of every five deaths in the United States is caused by tobacco use.

-Smoking causes more deaths every single year than all of the following causes combined:

HIV

Illegal Drug Use

Alcohol Consumption

Motor Vehicle Accidents

Firearm Related Incidents

-More than ten times as many United States citizens have died prematurely from smoking cigarettes than have died in all the wars fought by the United States in its history.

-Smoking causes about 90% of all lung cancer deaths in men and women. More women die from lung cancer every single year than from breast cancer.

Let us give you just a few of the health problems that are caused by using tobacco products:

-Stroke

-Asthma

-Infertility

-Aneurysms

-Menopause

-Emphysema

-Lung Cancer

-Liver Cancer

-Heart Attack

-Tooth Decay

-Gum Disease

-Colon Cancer

-Osteoporosis

-Inflammation

-Cervix Cancer

-Heart Disease

-Larynx Cancer

-Kidney Cancer

-Bladder Cancer

-Crohn's Disease

-Type 2 Diabetes

-Pancreas Cancer

-Esophagus Cancer

-Rheumatoid Arthritis

-Respiratory Infections

-Cardiovascular Disease

-Decreased Bone Density

-Increased Blood Pressure

The biggest problem from using any form of tobacco is of course: **DEATH!**

Using tobacco products is one of the very worst things you could ever do to your health, and is guaranteed to make you fat, sick, and **DIE**. If you continue to use tobacco you will continue to be fat and sick, and you will eventually **DIE** from the side effects. If you want to become lean, sexy, and healthy you absolutely must eliminate tobacco from your life. This is 100% non-negotiable!

Chapter Ten:

Not Exercising.

Not exercising will make you fat and sick, and you will die prematurely compared to if you had been exercising regularly. The ONLY reason why you wouldn't be exercising on a regular basis is because of some type of an EXCUSE that you tell yourself.

The number one excuse that people make for not exercising is that they're too busy. They don't have time to exercise. That's a big, fat lie! We all have the same amount of time. However, the people who exercise regularly make better use of their time than people who don't exercise. If you don't make time to exercise, then you better start preparing to spend time in the hospital because that's where you're going to end up.

People make time for the things that they think truly matter in life. Once you end up in the hospital and see the consequences of not exercising, your perspective on the importance of exercising will change. Hopefully, you won't allow that to happen. I'll bet you didn't know that one out of every ten premature deaths in the world today is because of not exercising. As crazy as this sounds, not exercising kills almost the same amount of people that smoking does. Approximately 250,000 people die every single year from not exercising. All you have to do to stay out of this group is simply exercise for just 30 minutes, three times per week. That will do wonders for your health.

Researchers did 25 different studies on people who don't exercise, and compared the results with people who do exercise. Every single study confirmed that people who don't exercise have a higher risk of depression. If you don't exercise you're missing out on the healing effects of what exercise can do to improve mood disorders. Exercising regularly reduces anxiety, increases self-esteem, and treats depression better than any pharmaceutical drug ever could.

People who don't do any strength training actually age faster than people who do strength training. Exercising with resistance training will help preserve bone density as you get older, while those who don't do resistance training will experience a greater risk of osteoporosis and bone fractures. Aging adults who don't exercise tend to fall more frequently than adults who do exercise.

The U.S. Department of Health and Human Services says that people who don't exercise have a much higher risk of getting sick and contracting different diseases. These include heart disease, diabetes, colon cancer, and high blood pressure. In fact, you'll catch the flu, or the common cold more often if you don't exercise. The National Institutes of Health reports that exercising will increase how quickly your white blood cells work, it will prevent the growth of various sickness causing bacteria, and it will flush bacteria out of your body.

Lack of exercise affects the heart, lungs, blood sugar levels, joints, bones, muscles, and mood. It also increases your risk of getting cancer. Not exercising also affects your ability to control your weight. This is why people are so fat and sick.

One of the major risk factors for getting heart disease is not exercising. The heart is a muscle and it grows stronger with exercise and is able to pump blood to all parts of the body more effectively. Exercising regularly gives you the most benefit for preventing heart disease. Regular exercise also helps keep your arteries flexible, guaranteeing that you have good blood pressure.

Even though you might not feel like exercising, it's one of the best things you could do for painful joints. Regular exercise can reduce pain, and help you control your weight. However, not exercising will only make your condition worse. If you don't exercise you won't receive the benefits of strengthening your muscles around your joints.

Exercising regularly will also give you more energy throughout the day, and help you lose weight faster compared to not exercising. Let us give you just a few of the health problems that are caused by not exercising:

-Anxiety

-Obesity

-Diabetes

-Joint Pain

-Depression

-Osteoporosis

-Colon Cancer

-Hypertension

-Heart Disease

-Breast Cancer

-Prostate Cancer

The biggest problem from not exercising is of course: **DEATH!**

Not exercising is one of the very worst things you could ever do to your health, and is guaranteed to make you fat, sick, and **DIE**. If you continue to not exercise you will continue to be fat and sick, and you will eventually **DIE** from the side effects. If you want to become lean, sexy, and healthy you absolutely must start exercising in your life. This is 100% non-negotiable!

Chapter Eleven:

How To Fix It.

In this chapter we're going to tell you our top 10 tips to make you lean, sexy, and healthy. The information in this book can add many years to your life. You can't fully enjoy life if your health is failing you. Most people's bodies are extremely toxic, with the average person containing over forty pounds of toxicity in their colon. With our top 10 tips you'll be able to give yourself a full body cleanse, which will eliminate the illness, sickness, and disease living inside of your body.

The information we've shared with you in this book works. We know firsthand. If you want to lose weight, cure yourself of so-called incurable diseases, and live life to the fullest, pay attention right now!

1. **Stay away from sugar!** It is an absolute health destroyer. Sugar will make you fat, sick, and you will eventually die from the side effects.

2. **Stay away from dairy!** It is an absolute health destroyer. Dairy will make you fat, sick, and you will eventually die from the side effects.

3. **Stay away from wheat!** It is an absolute health destroyer. Wheat will make you fat, sick, and you will eventually die from the side effects.

4. **Stay away from HFCS!** It is an absolute health destroyer. HFCS will make you fat, sick, and you will eventually die from the side effects.

5. **Stay away from drugs!** They are an absolute health destroyer. Drugs will make you fat, sick, and you will eventually die from the side effects.

6. **Stay away from alcohol!** It is an absolute health destroyer. Alcohol will make you fat, sick, and you will eventually die from the side effects.

7. **Stay away from tobacco!** It is an absolute health destroyer. Tobacco will make you fat, sick, and you will eventually die from the side effects.

8. **Start exercising immediately!** Not exercising is an absolute health destroyer. Not exercising will make you fat, sick, and you will eventually die from the side effects.

9. **Start eating organic food only!** Not eating organic food is an absolute health destroyer. Not eating organic food will make you fat, sick, and you will eventually die from the side effects.

10. **Start relaxing and having fun!** Not relaxing and having fun is an

absolute health destroyer. Not relaxing and having fun in life will make you fat, sick, and you will eventually die from the side effects.

Life is very short! You can probably remember where you were and what you were doing twenty years ago like it was just yesterday. We know we sure can. Life passes most people by and before they know it they're on their death bed wishing they would have, could have, and should have done more with their life. Well, the bad news is you only get to live life once, but the good news is as long as you're still alive it's not too late. Get started now! Stop making excuses and start taking action!

We can lead the horse to the water, but we can't make him drink.

To add even more value to this book we're going to give you our exact daily nutritional regimen and our weekly workout program for you to follow if you choose to. You don't have to follow our nutritional regimen if you don't want to, but if you do it will clean out all of the illness, sickness, and disease that is currently living inside of you. Our nutritional and workout regimens will help you become lean, sexy, and healthy faster than you can imagine.

As soon as we wake up in the morning:

We swallow 1 tbs of Coconut Oil.

We swallow 2 capsules of Korean Ginseng.

We gulp down ¼ cup of Apple Cider Vinegar.

We then drink our fat melting Hot Chocolate, which contains:

2 tbs of Cacao Powder.

4 tbs of Raw Honey.

1 tsp of Ground Cinnamon.

1 tsp of Ground Turmeric.

1 tsp of Ground Nutmeg.

1 tsp of Ground Ginger.

Thirty minutes after we wake up in the morning we go to the gym and do our cardio and resistance training on an empty stomach. We both cover ourselves in sweats and drink one can of sugar free Monster during our workouts.

We eat an Intermittent Fasting lifestyle for all our meals. We eat all our food between 2pm-10pm.

Meal 1 at 2:00 pm:

2 tbs of Flaxseed.

2 tbs of Chia Seeds.

1 serving of fresh fruit.

1 cup of Gluten Free Oatmeal.

Mix all ingredients in a bowl with hot water.

Meal 2 at 5:00 pm: protein shake.

2 tbs of Cacao Powder.

3 scoops of Raw Protein Powder.

16 ounces of Unsweetened Vanilla Almond Milk.

Mix all ingredients in a blender.

Meal 3 at 8:00 pm:

8 ounces of Lean Meat and tortilla chips seasoned with Cayenne Pepper.

Before we go to sleep at night:

We drink our fat melting Hot Chocolate, which contains:

2 tbs of Cacao Powder.

4 tbs of Raw Honey.

1 tsp of Ground Cinnamon.

1 tsp of Ground Turmeric.

1 tsp of Ground Nutmeg.

1 tsp of Ground Ginger.

We also drink one gallon of water filled with lemons every single day. This gives us energy, helps us lose bodyfat, and strengthens our immune systems. Drinking lemon water has all kinds of amazing health benefits. We highly encourage you to start drinking lemon water every single day. It will take your body from acidic to alkaline and can cure all kinds of illness, sickness, and disease.

Monday: Chest, Shoulders & Triceps.

Seated Chest Press: 3 sets by 20, 15, 12 (add weight each set).

Seated Shoulder Press: 3 sets by 20, 15, 12 (add weight each set).

Seated Tricep Press: 3 sets by 20, 15, 12 (add weight each set).

Wednesday: Quadriceps, Hamstrings, Glutes & Calves.

Seated Leg Press: 3 sets by 20, 15, 12 (add weight each set).

Seated Leg Curl: 3 sets by 20, 15, 12 (add weight each set).

Seated Leg Extension: 3 sets by 20, 15, 12 (add weight each set).

Leg Press Calf Raises: 3 sets by 20, 15, 12 (add weight each set).

Friday: Back, Biceps & Forearms.

Lat Pulldown: 3 sets by 20, 15, 12 (add weight each set).

Seated Row: 3 sets by 20, 15, 12 (add weight each set).

Seated Curls: 3 sets by 20, 15, 12 (add weight each set).

Monday: 20 minutes of interval based walking. Walk very quickly for 1 minute, then walk very slowly for 1 minute. You do this for 20 minutes.

Wednesday: 20 minutes of interval based walking. Walk very quickly for 1 minute, then walk very slowly for 1 minute. You do this for 20 minutes.

Friday: 20 minutes of interval based walking. Walk very quickly for 1 minute, then walk very slowly for 1 minute. You do this for 20 minutes.

You can substitute another form of cardio for walking if you want to. Switch it up and do the treadmill one day, the stationary bike one day, and the elliptical one day. That's three different cardio workouts per week. Every 20 minute cardio session you complete you're getting closer to your ultimate health goal.

We just gave you everything you need to know in order to become lean, sexy, and healthy. Now, you have to be the one who walks it out. If you start living by the information in this book you will add many years to your life. You'll have more energy, you'll be sexier, you'll be happier, and you'll be healthier. Who wouldn't want that? We hope and pray that you'll take action on what you've just read. When your health transforms please tell us about your success!

After you read this book would you mind doing us a huge favor please? Would you be kind enough to write us a five star customer review for this book on Amazon? By giving this book a good review it will help us as an author and help this book move up the rankings on Amazon. Your words have power. If you wouldn't mind supporting this book we would be extremely grateful. We would love to hear your feedback. You're welcome to contact us at our personal website anytime. If you would appreciate us sending you our self-publishing cheat sheet **ABSOLUTELY FREE**, just submit your name and email address at the link below. We wish you the very best of success in every area of your life!

Christopher & Stacy Mitchell

www.ChangeYourLifeOvernight.com

If you enjoyed reading this book here's more books by the authors:

1. How To Lose Weight With Intermittent Fasting!

2. Sell Your First Book!

3. The #1 How To Get Rich Book For Christian Men & Women!

4. My Inspiring True Life Story!

5. How To Get Rich From Home On A Part Time Basis With Only $20!

6. Minuscule To Muscular!

7. Faith Produces Miracles!

8. How To Make Money As An Author Selling Your Books On Amazon.

9. Money Meditation Manifestation!

All books can be purchased from:
www.ChangeYourLifeOvernight.com